I0425661

Vegan Diet for beginners: Easy, Delicious, healthy

An easy guide to becoming a vegan and living a healthier life.

Introduction

I want to thank you and congratulate you for downloading the book, *"Beginner's Guide to Veganism"*.

This book contains all the information you need to understand what veganism is, how to maintain health without animal products, and the environmental benefits of a vegan diet.

Veganism is not a hobby, nor should it be taken lightly. There are many health benefits to becoming a vegan, but if not done correctly, can lead to adverse health effects. This book will teach you how to not only enjoy a lifestyle free of animal products, but also how to do it safely.

It will also teach you all about the various other benefits of veganism, such as environmental effects and non-contribution to a cruel system of animal abuse.

Once you understand how easy veganism can be, how to do it healthily and the beneficial effects your diet has on the world around you, you'll wonder why you waited so long!

Thanks again for downloading this book, I hope you enjoy it!

Chapter 1 – What is Veganism?

You probably already know the basic tenets of veganism and how it is different from vegetarianism. Vegetarians abstain from eating meat and fish, while vegans take it a step further and eschew animal products in all shapes and forms, from food to clothing.

This means that to follow a truly vegan lifestyle – it is a lifestyle more than just a diet – you cannot eat meat, fish or poultry, nor any food or drink that is derived from animals. Similarly, using products or wearing clothing made from animal fibers or hides is against the definition of veganism.

There are different sorts of vegans, from those who subsist on natural plants to those who eat a lot of junk food (we'll get into the surprisingly long list of vegan junk food in a later chapter).

Similarly, there are many different reasons why one would go vegan. From preventing cruelty to animals as much as possible to the environmental benefits to health benefits, the reasons for going vegan are as different as vegans themselves. Indeed, there are many health benefits to going vegan, just as there are environmental benefits. The largest unifying factor among vegans, however, is that they disagree with the use of animals for the gain of humans.

We've all seen the stereotypes of the "annoying vegan" who proselytizes and chastises friends and strangers for eating animal products, but the truth is, it simply isn't true. Like many "annoying" subcultures, it's simply that the loudest proponents of a cause are those that get remembered.

The truth is, many vegans do it for personal reasons and it's really not necessary to sign up for militant converting duty in order to be a "good vegan". For many people, perhaps you included, choosing to follow a vegan lifestyle is a personal choice and has no bearing on other people.

If this diet and lifestyle is for you, be warned that it won't be easy. There are many people in the world who have unfounded prejudice against vegans. Stick with it, learn as much as you can and you will find that the rewards far outweigh the negative aspects.

Chapter 2 – History of Veganism

The diet known as veganism was first widely recognized in the 1940s due to a burgeoning group known as The Vegan Society. This society is still going strong, and is a great resource for navigating the ins and outs of becoming a vegan, not to mention keeping up with the latest news and initiatives.

The Society came up with a definition for veganism in 1949, including that their goals were to emancipate animals from the exploitation of humans. This involved not only abstaining from eating them or their products, but also advocating against hunting, use in medical or scientific research and use of animals for domestic chores.

These are very lofty goals, and it's obvious that they haven't been universally adopted. However, the adherence of vegans to their lifestyle means that there will always be those who value the existence of animals past their use for humans.

The Vegan Society has also coined three different phrases to represent the different motives and goals of vegans.

Dietary Vegans – Dietary vegans tend to focus on the health benefits of a vegan lifestyle. They don't partake in any animal products in their diet, but may use animal products such as wool. The ethical reasons are still there, but in general they aren't the main focus.

Ethical Vegans – Ethical vegans are just what the name suggests. They choose not to use anything made from animals, from food to clothing to labor. This is less for health reasons and more because they see the use of animals in any way to be a heinous exploitation. Very often, ethical vegans are the strictest when it comes to the use of animals and animal products.

Environmental Vegans – Environmental vegans choose to live an animal-free life for yet a different reason. Their personal philosophy often centers around the idea that using animals is harmful to the environment. From the factories necessary to the mass-production of meat for consumption to the questionable practices surrounding their farming, environmental vegans believe that by reducing our reliance on animals and their byproducts we can begin to practice more sustainable methods of supporting ourselves.

These three types of veganism may seem far removed from the initial aims and goals of The Vegan Society, but in reality they are just more specialized definitions. This way, all vegans are included and can find the niche to which they best identify.

Of course, if you don't identify as any of these three types of vegans, that's okay! The beauty of a vegan lifestyle is that as long as you follow its tenets you can choose your own reasons for doing so. It's a very inclusive community dedicated to helping others figure out their vegan identities.

Chapter 3 – Maintaining Health as a Vegan

The vegan lifestyle can be quite difficult to navigate – what's okay to eat or use, what isn't, what falls into a grey area? These are questions that just about all vegans have asked themselves at one point or another.

Not eating meat or fish, staying away from eggs and dairy as well as honey are pretty well-known aspects of being a vegan, but what else? Why is it important to veganism to not eat eggs or drink milk when it doesn't mean the animal has to be killed?

The reason is, even though you don't kill a cow for milk (and therefore all dairy products, including yogurt, cheese and butter) the same way you would for a steak or beef, it feeds the exploitation machine of animals. The majority of dairy cows are kept in a permanent state of lactation, which can be painful for the cow. It also means that they have calves who are almost immediately taken away from their mothers in order to provide more milk for human consumption.

The same goes for other animals. Chickens kept for laying purposes generally live in horrible conditions. While it is a natural process for a chicken to lay unfertilized eggs (the kind we eat), most vegans agree that we as humans don't have the right to exploit that for our own gain.

A lot of non-vegans may argue that because dairy cows and laying chickens aren't killed for their meat it's ethical to consume the other foods they produce. This argument, while logical on the surface, ignores the fact that these animals *are* being hurt. They are kept in terrible conditions, fed hormones to increase their production and subjected to lives of plain servitude.

Another argument non-vegans employ is that with a vegan diet it's impossible to get the necessary nutrients and vitamins to lead a healthy life. This is almost laughable, especially with the increasing popularity of plant-based protein in our society.

As many ancient cultures figured out long before the Western world, it's entirely possible to get the iron and protein your body needs without the sacrifice of animals. While you may be thinking you can only eat tofu and sprouts for the rest of your life, the real truth is that these days, it's possible to have a varied and delicious diet containing all the nutrients you need – and all vegan!

If you are worried that you aren't getting the nutrients and vitamins that you need, it's a simple procedure to visit your doctor and request bloodwork. That will let you know what, if anything, you are deficient or low in so you can take the proper steps to incorporate more in your diet. Let's look at the most important parts of anyone's diet.

Protein

Of all the dietary concerns associated with being a vegan, obtaining sufficient protein has to be the biggest. When we think of protein, we instinctively think of meat and fish and animal products. The truth is, there are a ton of different sources of protein to choose from at your local supermarket.

Tofu is probably the most well-known source of protein available. Its popularity in the west is surging, likely due to the fact that it has a bland flavor and inoffensive texture, making it ideal for a variety of different recipes. It can take on different seasonings and is as delicious in tacos or lasagna as it is in Asian cuisine.

For those craving a change, seitan and tempeh offer a far different texture from tofu. They're both made of soy as well, so you get a high amount of protein. These are similar to tofu in that they can be prepared in many different ways, but have a chewier texture and stronger flavor. If you've never tried them before, do so! They may become your new favorites.

Legumes are also a fantastic source of protein. Black beans, chickpeas and lentils are a vegan's best friend. Not only are they fantastically cheap, but easy to prepare and taste great. Environmental vegans love them because the production of these beans is far more sustainable and ecologically responsible than the raising of livestock. One of the best part of eating a diet rich in legumes? You can find thousands and thousands of recipes online – not all of them vegan, but with a little substitution you'll find that you can eat lentils every day of the week and never repeat a meal!

For a protein fix on the go, a handful of nuts is great. Peanuts and almonds contain a ton, so be sure to keep a baggie handy for that midday slump.

Fat

You may not think of fat as something you want a lot of in your diet, but for vegans it's important to get a good amount every day. The health risks of eating too little fat are magnified in a diet like veganism, as the majority of vegetables and fruits don't have much. Not having enough fat in your diet could lead to difficulties absorbing necessary vitamins, as well as leave you feeling unsatisfied.

Nuts have a fair amount of fats, as do avocado and seeds like flaxseed and chia seed. For many vegans, the growing popularity of coconut oil (and its subsequent presence in most grocery stores) is a godsend, as it is ridiculously versatile, delicious and contains a ton of health benefits despite its high fat content.

You may find that you have to take a supplement. If this is the case, opt for an Omega-3 supplement. Omega-3 fats have been found to prevent things like heart disease and dementia, so be sure to keep your levels at a good place!

Iron

The main culprit of the dreaded anemia is a lack of iron or difficulty absorbing iron. One of the biggest arguments you'll encounter as a vegan is that the best way to get adequate iron is to eat a lot of meat.

This simply is not true. In fact, you can get a ton of iron from a vegan diet if you eat the right foods. Don't avoid whole grains. Many people talk about the detriments of bread, pasta and the like, but whole grains are a great source of iron. So are legumes, so keep eating those beans and nuts! In fact, legumes are the superfood of the vegan diet as they are rich in iron, protein, good fats and myriad other vitamins necessary for good health.

One of the best ways to get a lot of iron in your diet is to eat foods rich in Vitamin C. These foods increase your body's ability to absorb and use the iron you take in. Vitamin C-rich foods include citrus, leafy greens and cauliflower.

If you find that you still aren't getting enough iron in your diet, supplements are very easy to come by and will give you all that you need!

Carbohydrates

Carbs get a bad rap, but that's mostly due to the prevalence of refined starches and carbs in our Western diet. In fact, carbs are a great addition to any diet. Not only do they provide you with energy that lasts a long time, but they can also help stabilize blood sugar – if you eat the right ones.

Stay away from white rice, refined flour, white potatoes and processed, carb-heavy or starchy foods. Instead, try to incorporate yams and sweet potatoes into your diet, as well as brown rice, grains like barley or quinoa, and bread made from unprocessed, unrefined flour.

If you feel like you can't eat enough of these foods, not to worry! Legumes and veggies also carry a bunch of carbs, so chances are this is the nutrition category you need to worry about the least.

Supplements

The majority of vegans take supplements of some sort in order to help them feel their best. While arguments that you can get all your necessary vitamins and nutrients simply by eating a whole diet, this is rarely the case. With all the scientific advances in vitamin supplements these days, as well as easy tests to determine which you are deficient in, the case for taking supplements is stronger than ever.

A B12 supplement is by far one of the most necessary. It's nigh impossible to get the optimum amount of B12 from a vegan diet alone, so please talk to your doctor about the recommended dose for you and the best way to take it.

Similarly, we talked about iron supplements. Not all vegans need these, but most do. Iron is a very important vitamin. It helps you feel energetic, healthy and stimulates good blood flow. These supplements are available over the counter at most grocery stores and drug stores, though if you have severe anemia your doctor may recommend a prescription supplement. Iron is especially important for women, as deficiencies are higher.

Calcium is another important supplement for women. True, eating heaps of cooked green vegetables will give you a fair amount, but who eats four cups of broccoli or kale per day? Many foods are fortified with calcium these days, but depending on personal preference, many vegan women find that they simply do not get enough. It may not matter as much to young people, but a persistent calcium deficiency can lead to severe health problems later in life, especially osteoporosis.

The takeaway

Try to get as many vitamins as you can from whole foods, but if you do need to take supplements, don't hesitate. They have so many health benefits and are way better for you than a diet rich in meat. In fact, many omnivores also take vitamins and supplements. A popular vegan argument is that they are akin to "cheating", but when it comes to your health and your values, it's important not to compromise.

Junk food

Junk food and processed vegan foods are very tempting. They're tasty, easy and convenient. Add to that the fact that a huge amount of popular snacks are "accidentally vegan" and it becomes ridiculously easy to lead a vegan life that isn't all that healthy.

As with an omnivorous diet, junk food is okay – in moderation. It's when it becomes the bulk of your diet that health issues such as vitamin deficiency, obesity and susceptibility to disease become apparent. Indulge, but sparingly.

As promised, here is a list of vegan junk food:

- Doritos (the Spicy Sweet Chili flavor)

- Most flavors of Kettle Brand Potato Chips

- Most flavors of Triscuits

- Oreos

- Wheat Thins

- Nature Valley Granola Bars

- Swedish Fish

- Thomas' Bagels

- Minute Maid Frozen Juice Bars

- Jell-O Instant Pudding

This isn't an exhaustive list, but they are among the most popular junk foods that are vegan-friendly (even if that wasn't their initial objective). As previously stated, you can subsist on Oreos and Triscuits alone and still be a vegan, but it is far from healthy.

A popular thing non-vegans say is that a vegan diet is all about sacrificing flavor and "good food". As you can see, this is far from the case. Moderation is key, but a vegan diet doesn't have to mean you can't indulge every now and then with one of your old favorites!

If you aren't sure whether your favorite chips or candy are vegan, a quick Google search will help you out. With veganism on the rise, there is no shortage of online lists of vegan foods. It's best to be safe, however, and check the ingredients.

When purchasing packaged or processed foods you should always check the ingredients first. There are a lot of different common ingredients that don't sound like they're made from animal byproducts that actually are.

The most famous one is gelatin. Many vegans (and even vegetarians) go a long time without realizing that gelatin is actually an animal product. It's prevalent in many different snacks, even Altoids!

Other things to watch out for:

- Albumen, which is derived from egg whites and present in a lot of packaged baked goods, as well as some wines.

- Bone meal, which is often found in calcium supplements, so be on the lookout for this scary ingredient!

- Casein, or caseinate is a milk protein. It's often found in non-dairy creamers or "vegan" cheese, making it not very vegan at all.

- Glycerin or glycerol are generally derived from animal fats and are prevalent in a wide variety of foods and other products.

- Lactose comes from animal milk and can be found in a variety of packaged baked goods.

- Rennet comes from cow stomachs and is used in wide array of foods.

As with the list of vegan junk food, this is by no means complete, merely the most commonly used animal derivatives found in food. There is an even longer list used in cosmetics and hygiene products, as well as medical supplies and medications.

While this isn't a complete set of information, it is to be hoped that it can help you make the best, most informed choices when it comes to following a vegan diet. Remember, it's possible to be incredibly healthy and vegan, but it takes dedication and study. Many common ingredients whose names give no indication they come from animals are actually animal products. Always read labels, talk to your doctor about the importance of abstaining from animal products, and don't be afraid to make dietary considerations known when you aren't cooking for yourself.

Chapter 4 – Environmental Benefits of Veganism

Even the most hardcore of meat eaters can't deny that adopting a diet free of meat and dairy products would have a substantial impact on the environment. In fact, a vegan diet helps protect our world by reducing pollution, limiting the effects of climate change and lessening the destruction of not only rain forests but other wooded areas.

Many vegans choose their lifestyle not because they feel eating meat is wrong (though most definitely do feel that way), but because they don't want to contribute to the destruction of an earth that their children and future descendants will inherit. It's more of an ecologically ethical issue than anything for them.

In fact, as long ago as 2010, the UN recommended that humans adopt a meat and dairy free diet not because they care about animals, but because they care about people. According to their studies, the impact that raising animals for food has on our environment is larger than ever, due in no small part to rising populations and rising demand for a meat-heavy diet.

How does a vegan diet reduce global warming? It's estimated that up to 20% of all greenhouse gases (the stuff that is heating up our earth) are produced by farmed livestock for human consumption. By reducing or eliminating altogether the raising of cows, chickens and pigs for food (as well as dairy cows and laying hens), the dire state of our climate would be drastically improved.

It's also estimated that the greenhouse gases produced by livestock are greater in volume than that of every mode of transportation in use today. Simply raising a cow for slaughter has more impact on climate change than driving a car everywhere!

With the population of the earth expected to reach 9 billion in just 35-40 years, and assuming a constant rate of meat and dairy consumption, this problem is only going to get worse.

One major concern is space. Livestock (especially cattle) require a massive amount of room to live. This, combined with growing population, means that there is less land available for more sustainable food sources such as grains, legumes and produce. The sad fact is, everyone needs to eat. And as long as the majority of people are clamoring for cheeseburgers and milkshakes, more and more land will be set aside for the cruel, destructive practice of raising animals for our exploitation.

By switching grazing land to grain or legume fields, it not only decreases the amount of greenhouse gases emitted, but also yields a much higher volume of nutritious food per acre. This is much more sustainable and more likely to handle the food demands of an exploding global population. In addition, with less livestock being farmed, more of the grains and legumes grown around the world can be consumed by the hungry. With all of our resources and technological advances, there should be no reason for people to go hungry. A vegan diet is a stance against the greed and avarice of our society.

The space required to house livestock contributes to another heinous crime against our earth – the felling of large swathes of wooded area. Logging has always been a contentious subject, but many countries around the world have laws in place that state that all trees felled for commercial use must be replaced with seedlings or saplings.

This is sadly not the case when land that used to be home to a wide variety of biodiversity is now taken over solely for the raising of cattle. The lack of trees is bad for the environment, but it also displaces a large array of other animals, forcing them into urban areas or sentencing them to death.

In the fish industry, demand for fish has led to some pretty gruesome consequences. The most famous are the cruelty toward dolphins and whales as well as the overfishing of tuna, but what about the effect that has on the oceanic ecosystem?

For caught fish, overfishing leads to an imbalance of predators and prey in the oceans. The majority of fish we eat falls somewhere in the middle, eating smaller fish and being eaten by larger ones. When we reduce fish populations to a shadow of their former selves, smaller fish are able to thrive, in turn decimating the population of those smaller than themselves. Larger fish generally do not go after them as it's not in their instincts. Human demand for fish has literally wrought havoc on the food chain.

As for farmed fish, one of the biggest issues is farming non-native species. No matter how safe or contained a fish farm is, escapes happen. While it's a heart-warming image of a little fish destined to become sushi escaping captivity, there are negative effects.

One of the biggest is the impact on the native populations. Introduced fish can carry diseases that native fish have never been exposed to, leading to death in epidemic-like numbers. Many people who eat fish simply have no idea of the impact their choices make. Indeed, most vegetarians and vegans don't realize it either.

The detriments of the fishing industry are not as picturesque or as easy to relate to as those of the livestock industry. Awareness is growing, but slowly.

If the environment and health and safety of the world around you is important to you, the best defense you have is to tell the meat and fish industry that you will not contribute to the destruction of our earth and most precious resources.

Chapter 5 – Ethical Reasons for Veganism

By far the majority of vegans choose their lifestyle because they cannot face contributing to an industry that systematically harms animals. They also feel that they have no right to exploit defenseless creatures for their own gain.

You may feel like animal's rights and human rights go hand in hand, which is fairly common. After all, like us, the animals we kill and eat are capable of emotions. They feel pain and they feel fear (even fish!), and many people cannot bring themselves to inflict that (or contribute to it) on another living animal.

However, the ethical reasons for going vegan are deeper than that.

We all know about the shocking videos online, those taken inside slaughterhouses and chicken pens. These are major reasons for vegetarians to eschew meat and animal byproducts. And yet, they feel comfortable eating eggs and cheese and drinking milk.

The truth is, many dairy farms kill male calves as soon as they are born. Their inability to produce milk makes them useless in the eyes of an industry focused on profits, therefore they are simply culled. The same goes for male chicks in laying houses.

As for the elderly dairy cows and laying hens, once their production starts to decrease, they are seen as a burden. Even if they are still producing, if it isn't at optimal levels, they aren't worth the cost to feed and house. They are also culled, even if they are healthy enough to live for years after.

One reason ethical vegans don't eat honey is because whole hives are sometimes culled after honey is harvested! Bees don't make their honey for humans to eat, they make it for themselves. When it's taken from them, many work themselves to death to rebuild stocks, which are then harvested again.

We may think that just because we aren't killing an animal to eat its flesh, it's okay to use them. It isn't. Many are killed anyway for selfish purposes. All are exploited in some manner.

For all of these reasons, many people choose to identify as ethical vegans.

Chapter 6 – Veganism Goes Beyond Food

Adhering to a vegan lifestyle is about more than just the food you eat. It involves eschewing all animal products entirely.

It's obvious that leather and other hides are not part of a vegan lifestyle, as animals must die for their production, but did you know that fibers such as angora, silk or wool are also not vegan? Although the animals needn't die for these fabrics to be produced, it is still a form of exploitation, which is why many vegans choose to wear synthetic fibers.

Of course, if you have sensitivity to some synthetic fibers, plant fibers such as cotton, linen and hemp are among the most common when it comes to clothing. To be sure, finding vegan clothing is one of the easiest parts of embracing this lifestyle! Many faux leather alternatives look like the real thing, so if you're in it for aesthetic purposes, you don't have to sacrifice fashion. The same goes for fake fur. It looks fun and funky, without the ridiculous price tag that usually accompanies wearing animal skin.

In addition, animal byproducts are a prevalent ingredient in both cosmetics and hygiene products, not to mention medicines. This is separate from the issue of animal testing, which is also unsettlingly common in this day and age.

With all the technological advances available to us, there is simply no reason to continue testing cosmetics and medications on animals. The conditions in which they are kept create environments of pain and fear, not to mention the detrimental effects of chemicals on their bodies.

In order to spare as much pain and exploitation of animals as possible, opt for vegan-friendly options. They are easier to find than you would think, and many well known brands make it a point to provide ethical, vegan products.

Some of the more famous vegan cosmetics brands include Manic Panic, e.l.f. Studio Cosmetics, and the majority of Urban Decay products. If you're having difficulties finding exactly what you want from these companies, or the price is a bit too high (vegan cosmetics tend to be high-end), search labels for ingredients such as beeswax, lanolin, carmine, collagen and tallow.

It's also important to make sure that the brushes you use are vegan. Many are made from animal hair, such as boar bristles or mink fur. Luckily, it's pretty easy to find synthetic hair brushes these days. They do just as good a job, and are usually a fraction of the price!

As for hygiene products and skin care, it's a little more difficult to find affordable, vegan options.

Shampoo and conditioner are two of the biggest offenders in this. However, Nature's Gate and 100% Pure are solid options. For a more economical choice, the L'Oreal EverPure line is not only made without animal products, but is also not tested on animals, something the other major drugstore brands can't say.

It's a little harder to check the ingredients on hair products, as many might be derived from plants or animals, but it's best to stay on the safe side and go with proven vegan hair care.

Skin care is also a bit iffy. Not only is animal testing prevalent (even though they have very different skin from humans), but the ambiguous source of ingredients is the same as in hair care.

With that said, you cannot go wrong with anything from Lush (one of the best and most high-profile cruelty-free brands available), Yes To or 100% Pure. These companies are committed to bringing you great products without any harm to animals, a promise that is very valuable these days.

As for medications or other medical tools, it's best to talk to your doctor. While many medicines these days contain no animal products, some do, and a doctor will be best able to let you know which ones. The real issue comes from animal testing. The scientific and medical research fields are notorious for their use of animals in inhumane trials and testing. Again, it's difficult to know which were tested on animals, but speaking with your doctor and voicing your concerns is the best way to stay informed.

If you do have health issues that can best be treated with a non-vegan solution, remember that your health should be the most important thing to you. Maintaining a vegan lifestyle is amazing, but it should not compromise your physical or mental health in any way.

Chapter 7 – Dealing With a Vegan Lifestyle

One of the major obstacles vegans face in everyday life is the judgement of others. It comes from family, friends and even absolute strangers. So many people have negative preconceived notions about vegans, and it can be hard to overcome them.

Mentioning that you're a vegan is important; if you're dining with others, it gives them an idea of your dietary restrictions. If you're having an ethical debate, it's a hint of where your ideology lies. The sad truth is, many people take the mention of veganism to be proselytizing. Worse, they may think you are judging them and their dietary decisions.

The best way to counteract these stereotypes is to simply empathize. If you feel the need to sell the vegan lifestyle to others, it can be helpful to put yourself in their shoes. Think of aggressive door-to-door salesmen or religious zealots trying to gain converts. The stigma against veganism in our society is such that any mention of reasons for veganism is instantly taken in that vein.

Make it clear that your decisions are about you. They don't affect anyone else but you, and it's important to you that others understand this. Unfortunately, it may take a few tries as humans in general don't like to feel as though they are being judged. Many people, when you tell them you're a vegan, will think you believe yourself to be more moral. Whether or not that's the case, understand why people react the way that they do and either try to empathize or stop caring.

Honestly, giving up on caring what other people think of your habits and diet is one of the most freeing feelings in the world.

Your lifestyle is nobody's business but your own. You don't owe excuses or reasons to anyone but yourself. Remember that and you will be much happier.

Luckily, veganism is becoming much more mainstream. The majority of new converts are dietary vegans or those who care about the environment, but their prevalence (coupled with a strong celebrity presence) are helping to make veganism less "weird" and more an accepted personal choice.

The difference between vegan diet options now and just twenty years ago is staggering! Not only that, but the trouble food makers and restaurants go to when properly labeling ingredients has greatly improved. These days, you're just as likely to find a vegan muffin in your grocery store bakery as you are at the most hipster of coffee shops!

Going vegan, whether it's for dietary, environmental or ethical reasons, is no longer the hardship it used to be. It's becoming more widely accepted as a way of life, and with acceptance comes more widespread adoption.

Be proud of your choices, stay on top of your health, and always have a little snack handy in case you can't find something suitable when out and about.

Conclusion

Thank you again for downloading this book!

I hope this book was able to help you understand more about becoming a vegan.

The next step is to find out what veganism means to you, why you choose the lifestyle and how you can help make the world a better place for humans and animals alike.

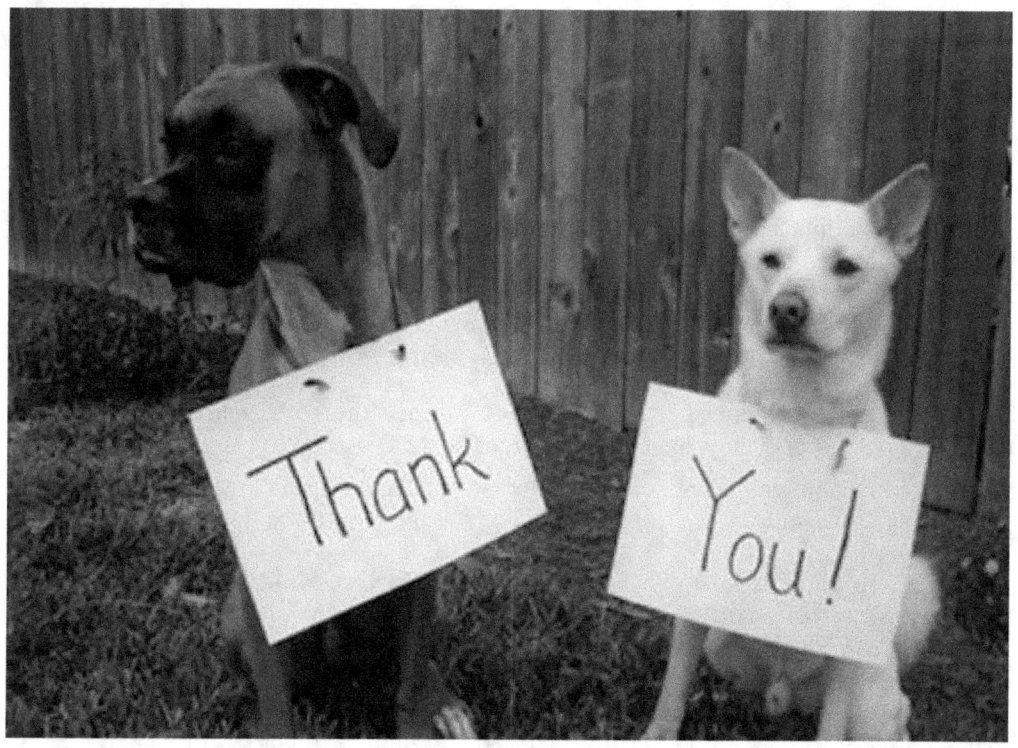

Finally, if you enjoyed this book, then I'd like to ask you for a favor, would you be kind enough to leave a review for this book on Amazon? It'd be greatly appreciated!

Thank you and good luck!

Chapter 4 – Caring for Organic Vegetables & Fruits

Depending on the plant varieties you choose, your organic vegetable or fruit garden will continue to yield edibles for months at a time. A large variety will also provide a ton of color and beauty.

A lot of the continuing care of your garden will depend on the variety of species you plant. Honestly, your choices are endless, but for brevity's sake, here are care guidelines for some of the more common fruit and veggie choices.

Vegetables

Beans are a popular choice. Green beans are easy to grow and can be harvested throughout the summer and early fall, making them a versatile and long-lasting crop. If space is a concern, grow pole beans. They grow vertically, so will require a stabilizing pole or trellis, but the crop to area ratio is amazing. They also require little in the way of fertilizer since they produce most of the nitrogen they need.

Plant beans in the spring, just after the last frost. The seedlings take well to slightly cooler soil temperatures and they have a growth period of 2-3 months, so start early. They require a moderate amount of sun and water, so special care isn't a necessity with these easy, versatile veggies.

Beets are also quite popular. They come in many varieties, all of which have different tastes and grow periods. Red table beets are by far the most common, as well as the easiest to grow. They do take a while to produce edible roots, so plant these guys a month or so before the last spring frost.

The good news is, they are very hardy. It's actually quite difficult to kill a good crop of beets, so these are a good choice for "black thumbs". They are also very versatile. While the root itself takes several months to reach an edible state, the greens can be harvested as soon as they reach a few inches long. Water them moderately and try to keep them out of harsh sunlight so as not to kill the greens.

For beauty as well as tastiness, why not try cabbage? Whether you choose green or red cabbage, you will be surprised at just how easy they are to grow. Not only are they delicious and nutritious whether cooked or raw, but they are absolutely gorgeous when growing.

One advantage is that you can harvest cabbage twice, once in the spring and again in the fall. These guys love a slight frost toward the end of their growth period, so don't worry about leaving them in the ground too late in the year. They require moderate water, but should be sheltered from too much sun. It is a good idea to do some research on how big each species will grow, and space the seedlings accordingly. Some cabbages can grow to massive proportions, so be careful they don't encroach on each other.

Carrots are always a good choice for a small garden. Chantenay carrots are by far the most popular, as well as one of the easiest to grow. They're the cone-shaped variety you find at the grocery store. Other varieties have different tastes and shapes, but many are a bit picky about where they grow and require a little more dedication.

Plant your carrots early, as they take a few months to get to the edible stage. They're best when planted in the spring, then harvested in summer and fall. The good news is that carrots do well with just about any type of soil, need only a little bit of sun and are fine with moderate watering. Carrots are surprisingly easy to grow and very difficult to kill, making them perfect for a starter garden.

Onions are a staple food around the world, and with so many different varieties, it's easy to find a species that grows perfectly in your climate. There are three types of onions, short-day, intermediate-day and long-day. The types correspond to the length of summer days they grow best in. For example, in the north, summer days last longer sunrise to sunset, so a long-day variety grows quite well.

Once you've chosen your onion variety, it's best to start the seedlings in the winter. Grow them in the house at first, then transfer them to the garden in the spring. These guys absolutely love a lot of sun, so don't be afraid to plant them in the sunniest spot you can find.

Harvest once the tops have fallen, and move them to a dry, shady spot for a few days until they're a little drier and ready to eat.

Peppers are an organic garden's darling. Not only are there a ton of different varieties to choose from, but they are very easy to take care of. You can grow bell peppers, sweet peppers or hot peppers. These will need a stabilizing pole or trellis of some sort, as the plants themselves are long and spindly, while the peppers tend to weigh them down a bit.

Peppers love warm weather, so start the seedlings inside, preferably in the early spring. Grow them until a few weeks after your last frost, then transfer them outside. For a few days before planting them in your garden, let them sit outside for a few hours each day. This way, they will become acclimated to the great outdoors and won't suffer culture shock when transplanted.

Peppers, while easy to care for, do need a lot of sun and water. It's best to keep them separated from root veg, as they require a lot more water and you don't want your carrots getting greedy!

You can harvest peppers as soon as you think they're big enough to eat, though the longer you leave them on the vine the more flavorful and full of vitamins they will be. Dried or pickled peppers will keep a long time, making these an excellent choice for canning.

Tomatoes are one of the most popular choices for home gardening. With so many varieties to choose from (including lovely heirloom types), you're guaranteed to find a species to love. One of the benefits of choosing organically grown tomatoes over the store bought kind is flavor! Store bought tomatoes have typically been genetically modified to look plump and juicy and bright red. Unfortunately, this results in a bland, almost mushy flavor. Your garden-grown tomatoes may not look perfect, but you'll taste the difference with the first bite.

Similar to peppers, you want to start them indoors in the early spring and transplant them around the same time. Acclimatize your tomato plants to the outdoors in the same way.

Because tomatoes need a lot of sun and water, they are great companion plants to peppers. Plant them in the same area and make sure they both get lots of sun and water throughout their growth. Also like peppers, tomatoes can be harvested as soon as you think they're ready, though it's best to leave them on the vine until they are at least a little red!

Fruits

Blueberries are a popular addition to an organic garden. You only need to look at how easily and profusely they grow in the wild to get an idea of how easy it will be to have fresh blueberries in your own garden!

Start blueberries indoors, preferably in the late winter, around January or February. The fruits are small, but the plants themselves need extra time to put down firm roots. Set them out a month or two after initial planting, before the really warm weather hits.

Once your blueberry plant is planted nice and deep and the roots have taken, they really need very little. A sunny patch, a little water and they grow like nobody's business all on their own.

One of the best aspects of growing berries is that they can be left on the bush for quite a while. Pull them off when you want some berries, pop some in your mouth when going about your gardening, and leave the big harvest for late summer. Blueberries are great for preserves and canning, so be sure to save some!

Grapes are a popular choice for trellis coverings, and with a large variety to choose from, it's easy to find one that is perfect for your climate. In general, it's easier to grow grapes in dry climates, but with a little extra care and direct sunlight, grapes can thrive even in humid areas.

For colder climates or those with shorter summers, choose white or green grapes. They ripen more quickly and their thinner skin means they thrive on less heat and sunlight. For longer summers or hotter weather, choose a darker grape. Their thicker skins can handle the intense heat.

Honestly, unless you're going for a prize-winning wine grape, you can grow delicious grapes with little interference. Because they are vine-grown, they do need a fence or trellis to grow along. Natural sunlight and a little water is best, though if you have moderate rain, that's sufficient for their growth. Larger, dark grapes are amazing for jam-making and juicing, while green or white grapes are particularly spectacular when eaten directly off the vine.

Strawberries are one of the most popular home-grown fruits. That's because they bear fruit very easily, are adaptable to different weathers and soil types and taste *so much better* than store bought varieties. Sure, most organically grown fruits and vegetables taste better than the grocery store equivalent, but with strawberries (like tomatoes) the difference is staggering.

For strawberries, it's recommended to start with small plants. You can plant seeds, but keep in mind that it will take one or two years before you start to see any edible fruits. Strawberry plants are not expensive, however, and you can plant seeds every year to have a renewable crop, as one plant will last three or four years by itself.

They love sunny patches, so be sure to keep them out of the shade. Strawberries do well when in the company of other berries, so if you have enough space, think about a mixed berry patch! They have similar growth patterns and needs to blueberries and blackberries, which means you will be up to your elbows in cobblers and jams in no time!

No matter what fruits or vegetables you decide to plant, just be sure that you read directions for planting and pay attention to the individual needs of each species. Once you have a starter garden planted and feel more confident in your gardening abilities, why not try out other, more exotic foods? Heirloom veg are beautiful and often have very unique flavors. Fruit trees, while they are a bit of a time commitment, are a lovely addition to any garden or lawn.

Find out what's best for your climate and soil and plan from there! You can enjoy foods fresh from the garden within a season.

Click HERE To read the full book

Other Books To Read

Below you'll find some other recommended books that are popular on Amazon and Kindle as well. Simply click on the links below to check them out.

Organic Gardening – A beginners step by step guide **by Lisa Shine**

Meditation: Powerful Guide to Meditation in Everyday Life

Cannabis & Cancer: The Medicinal benefits of this miracle herb

If the links do not work, for whatever reason, you can simply search for these titles on the Amazon website to find them.